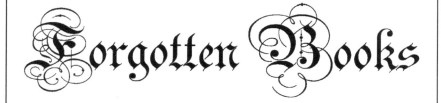

ISBN 978-0-428-14768-6
PIBN 11249575

1 MONTH OF
FREE
READING

at

www.ForgottenBooks.com

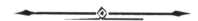

By purchasing this book you are eligible for one month membership to ForgottenBooks.com, giving you unlimited access to our entire collection of over 1,000,000 titles via our web site and mobile apps.

To claim your free month visit:

www.forgottenbooks.com/free1249575

English
Français
Deutsche
Italiano
Español
Português

www.forgottenbooks.com

Mythology Photography **Fiction**
Fishing Christianity **Art** Cooking
Essays Buddhism Freemasonry
Medicine **Biology** Music **Ancient
Egypt** Evolution Carpentry Physics
Dance Geology **Mathematics** Fitness
Shakespeare **Folklore** Yoga Marketing
Confidence Immortality Biographies
Poetry **Psychology** Witchcraft
Electronics Chemistry History **Law**
Accounting **Philosophy** Anthropology
Alchemy Drama Quantum Mechanics
Atheism Sexual Health **Ancient History**
Entrepreneurship Languages Sport
Paleontology Needlework Islam
Metaphysics Investment Archaeology
Parenting Statistics Criminology
Motivational

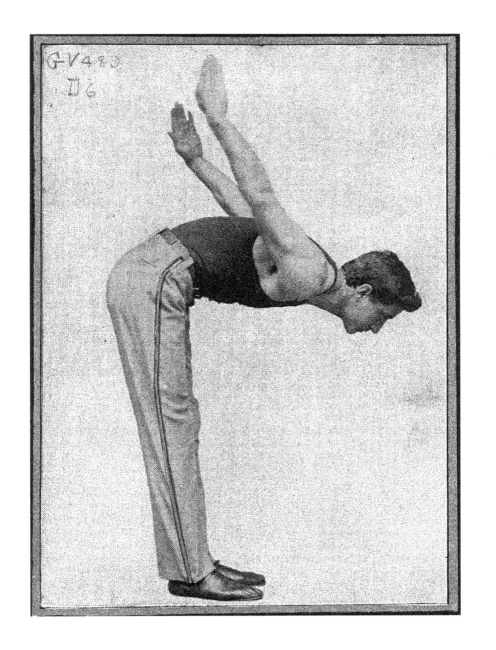

U. S. ARMY
PHYSICAL EXERCISES

REVISED FOR THE USE OF THE CIVILIAN

BY

PROFESSOR DONOVAN

Author of " The Art of Boxing and Self-Defense," etc.

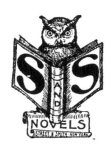

NEW YORK

STREET & SMITH, Publishers

238 William Street

Copyright, 1902
By STREET & SMITH

U. S. Army Physical Exercises

PREFACE..

The exercises which are here illustrated are taken from the Infantry Drill Regulations of the United States Army, but differ in one or two instances from the regular setting-up exercises, as they are called.

The various movements are practiced by all soldiers in garrison in order to retain a proper set-up and to keep the muscles supple; but they are essentially military in character, and I have made a few necessary changes so that the civilian who wishes to employ the exercises may reap the fullest benefit from their use.

The illustrations are from thirty original photographs posed expressly for this work by Prof. M. Chas. Benisch, Instructor of the Central Civil Science School and Gymnasium.

PROFESSOR DONOVAN.

CONTENTS.

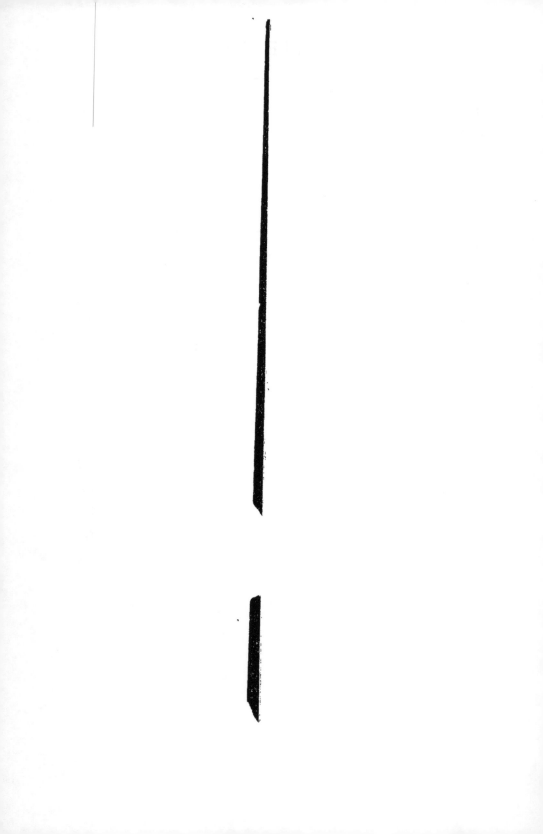

UNITED STATES ARMY

PHYSICAL EXERCISES.

SETTING-UP EXERCISES.

INTRODUCTION.

Exercise is an absolute necessity—as necessary to a proper existence as the air we breathe. Many people crawl through life but half-developed when the road to salvation in this respect is close at hand—that is, a regular course of scientific exercise every day. Any ordinary person who has not previously done any training, and is practically undeveloped, should be able to double his strength within twelve months by devoting from twenty minutes to half an hour twice daily to exercise.

As to the method of exercising, there is nothing better than the setting-up exercises of the U. S. Army, which are here illustrated and explained. They were designed especially for soldiers, "to keep the muscles supple and maintain an erect set-up." But they are equally suited to the civilian, and ought to be familiar to every person who values a strong and healthful body.

The best time to practice these setting-up exercises —which, by the way, are very simple and need no apparatus—is not the morning, but, rather, the afternoon or evening.

As a matter of fact, a man is precisely at his weakest when he turns out of bed in the morning. The muscular force is greatly increased by breakfast, but it attains to its highest point after the midday meal. It then sinks for a few hours, and rises again toward evening. Morning is absolutely the worst time for practice; the setting-up exercises, if used first thing, leave an effect, a tired feeling, which is felt for the rest of the day.

If most writers on physical culture agree that four o'clock is the best time for training, it is probably because the adoption of this time will have allowed at least two hours for the process of digestion to have taken place. Training either immediately before or directly after a meal should be strongly discou\-

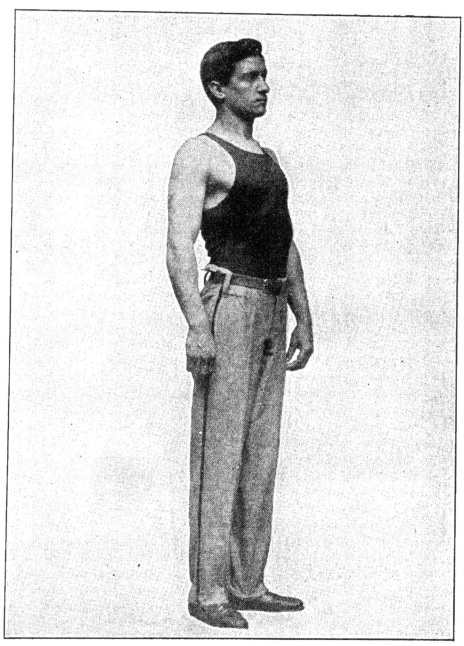

FIGURE 1.

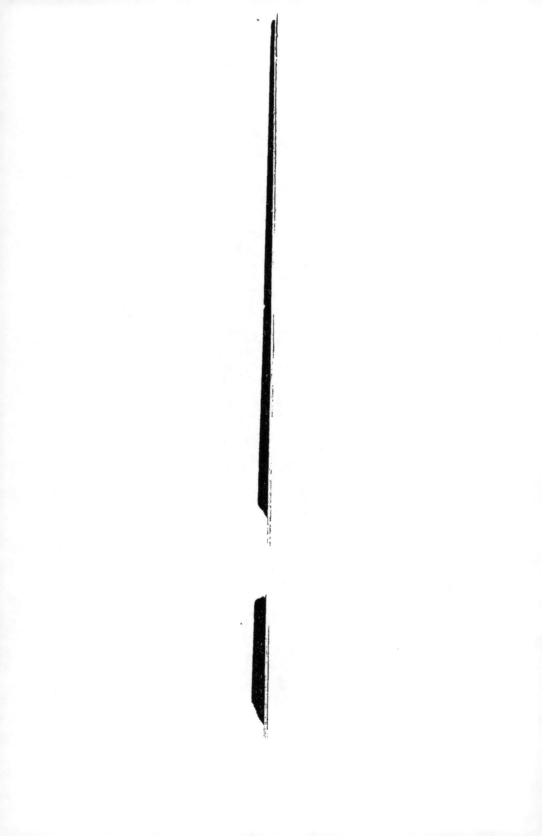

tenanced, the blood that is required for digestion being drawn to the muscles.

Care must be taken that the muscles are placed under the most favorable condition during exercise. Deep breathing should be practiced when exercising. After an inhalation the breath should be held for a second or two, and then slowly exhaled.

The room in which you exercise should never be dusty or ill-ventilated. All flexions or extensions should be deliberately and smoothly performed, with the mind strongly concentrated on the muscle or muscles affected.

The movements should be commenced rather quickly, and finished more gradually. Each movement should be repeated in the same time as the preceding one. While exercising, keep the power of recuperation always in mind.

Unless you have plenty of time, do not attempt to go through all the exercises at one time, but as far as you go, work thoroughly, and at the next opportunity for exercise commence where you left off. It is better to alternate the *arm, hand, trunk, leg* and *foot* exercises and interrupt the drill with occasional rests.

At first, when the novelty wears off, the training may grow to be considered irksome; but if the pupil will only persevere, in time the setting-up exercises will be found as necessary as a meal, and their cessation will be considered a deprivation.

To mark the gain in his development, the pupil should set down the date at which he commenced to practice, and take his height, weight and muscular measurements, and at stated intervals afterward register the increase he has gained as the result of exercise, and as an encouragement to progress.

It is much better to exercise a quarter of an hour a day regularly than to exercise for a couple of hours or more at a time at irregular intervals.

In fine weather, if you cannot exercise in the open air, throw open the window of your room, taking care that you are not in a draught. If possible, go through the exercises stripped to the waist.

At the finish of the exercises a good rub down with a rough towel or a very rough pair of flesh gloves should follow. The cold bath should be regularly taken some time during the day; just after exercise, is perhaps the best time. After the bath the body should be rubbed dry with a rough towel.

By following the instructions and rules here given, not only can the development of a clean, rounded and

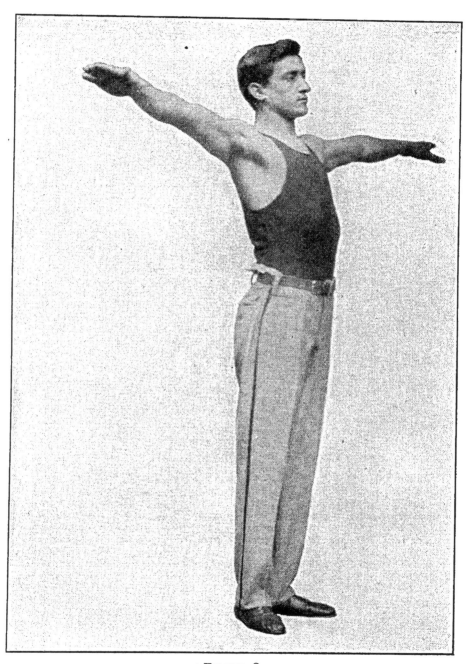

FIGURE 2.

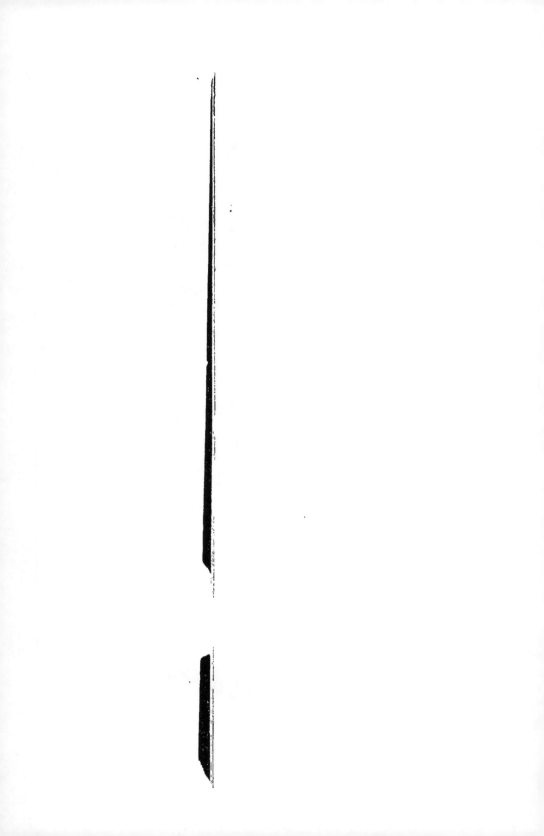

elastic form be anticipated, but the healthfulness of the practice will furnish a sound playground for geniality, good-nature and enjoyment, and you should be able to produce muscle that could be compared to a well-assorted arrangement of steel plates.

FIRST EXERCISE.

The military commands for this exercise are:

1. Arm.

2. Exercise.

3. Head.

4. Up.

5. Down.

6. Raise.

ARM.

1. Take the position as in figure 1, heels together, just touching the floor, toes turned outward, shoulders well back, chest forward, whole body inclined slightly to the front so that the greatest weight will rest on the balls of the feet.

EXERCISE.

2. Raise the arms from the sides to a horizontal position, with the palms downward.

See Fig. 2.

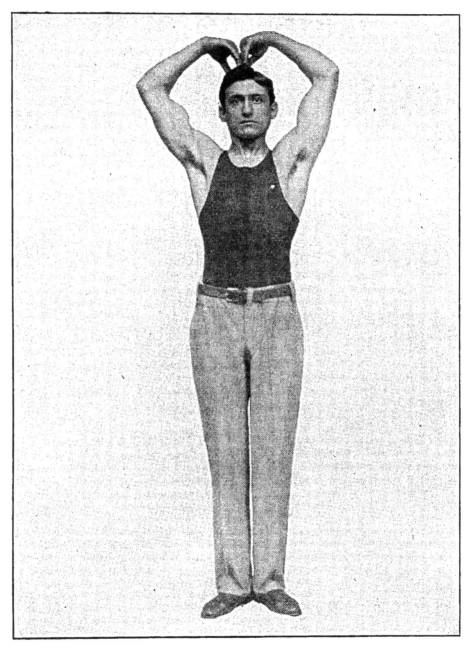

FIGURE 3.

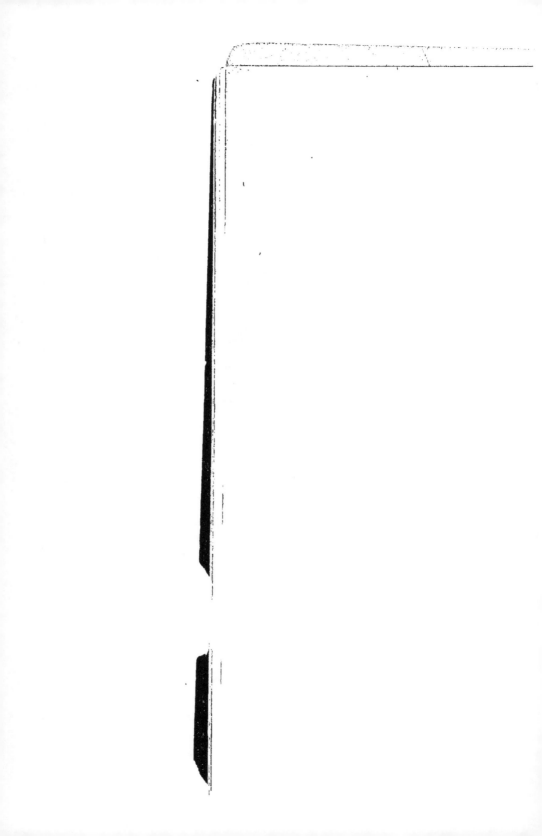

HEAD.

3. Raise the arms from the sides in a circular direction above the head, bending the forearm so that the tips of the fingers will meet and touch the head over the forehead.

The backs of the fingers should be in contact their full length from the moment they touch after the circular swing.

Keep the elbows pressed well backward.

The thumbs should point directly to the rear.

See Fig. 3.

UP.

4. Extend the arms upward their full length, with palms facing.

This exercise may be varied by bringing the palms close together over the head, the arms being kept rigid.

See Fig. 4.

DOWN.

5. Force the arms backward in an oblique direction, and gradually lower them to the sides of the thighs.

See Fig. 1.

RAISE.

6. Raise the arms sideward, as prescribed for the second command.

Continue exercise from 3 onward.

When two or more friends are exercising in company, one may, while resting, give the commands for each movement, recommencing with the word *raise*, and continuing by repeating *head, up, down, raise.*

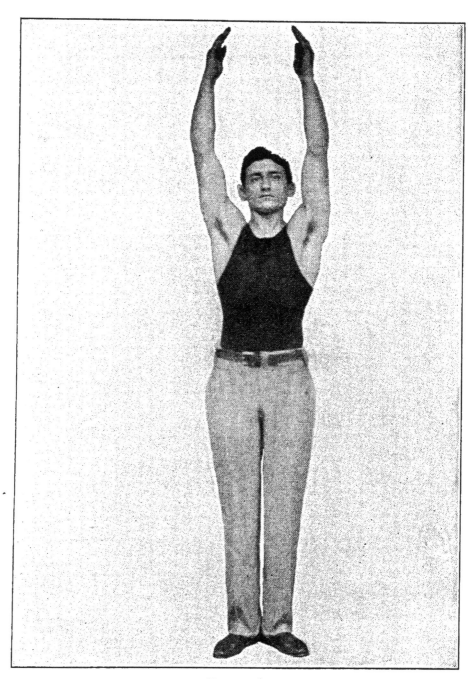

FIGURE 4.

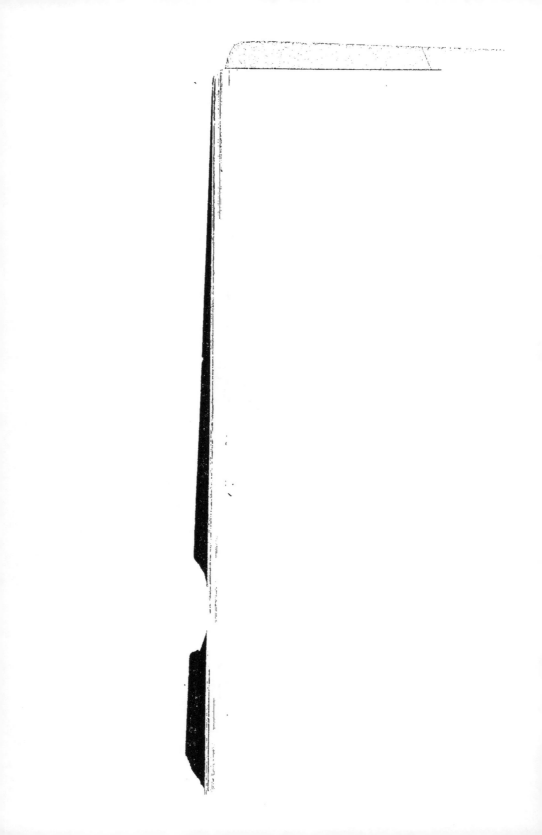

SECOND EXERCISE.

The military commands for the second exercise are:

1. Arm.

2. Exercise.

3. Front.

4. Rear.

ARM.

1. Take position as in Figure 1.

EXERCISE.

2. At the command *exercise,* raise the arms laterally, as directed in first exercise (see Figure 2).

FRONT.

3. Swing the arms, extended, from the sides horizontally to the front.

The palms should touch at the limit of the extension.

Do not rise on the toes.   Keep the heels on the ground.

See Fig. 5.

REAR.

4. Swing the extended arms with a rapid sweep from the front to the rear.

The arms on taking position at rear may have a slight downward inclination.

In the swing to the rear raise the heels from the ground, bearing the entire weight of the body on the toes.

See Fig. 6.

Continue the front and rear movements until able, if possible, to touch the hands behind the back.

In using commands repeat *front, rear,* for continuance of exercise.

Do not be half-hearted in this and similar exercises.

Put energy, life and determination into effort.

Be certain that every muscle possible is brought into play.

Only thus will the setting-up exercises be of any use.

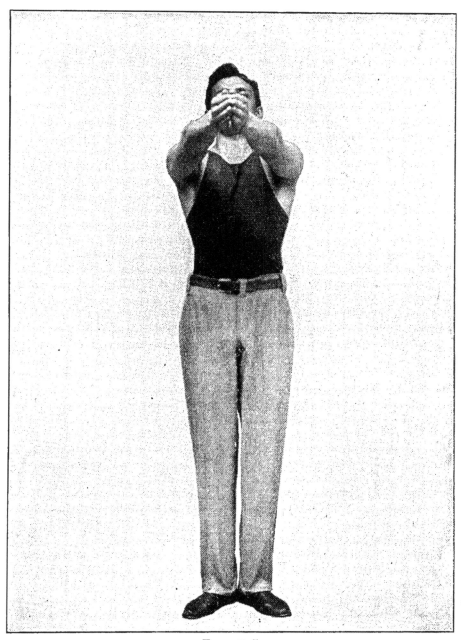

FIGURE 5.

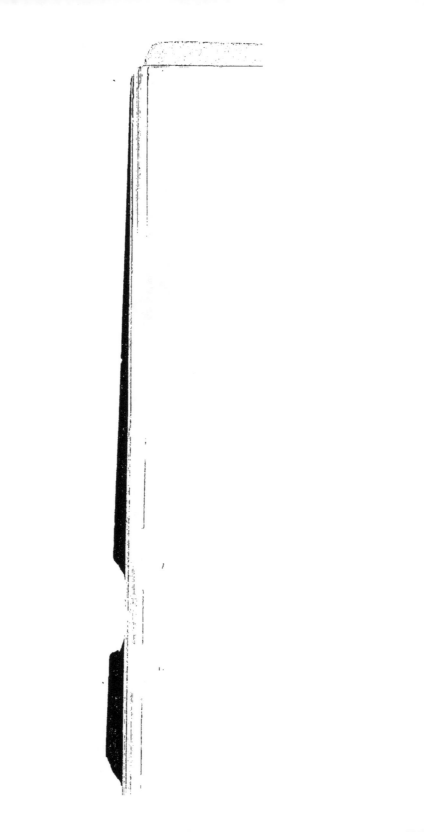

THIRD EXERCISE.

The military commands for the third exercise are:

1. Arm.

2. Exercise.

3. Circle.

ARM.

1. Position as in Figure 1.

EXERCISE.

2. At the command *exercise,* raise the arms from the sides, as in first exercise.

CIRCLE.

3. With each arm describe a circle upward and backward, on each side of the head.

Let the action in this instance be slow at first, and increasing only slightly as continued.

The arms should not pass in front of the line of the breast at any time during this exercise.

Keep the arms to the rear as much as possible.

See Fig. 7.

In using command simply repeat the word *circle* for continuance of exercise.

Do not return to second movement after completing the circle. Continue slowly to describe circles, commencing each time with the word *circle* if commands are used.

This is a very excellent exercise for developing the chest.

While making the circles, occasionally draw in a deep inhalation and retain it while two or three motions are made, before expelling.

This tends to force out the walls of the chest more thoroughly, and thus gives room for the process of enriching the blood with those elements that build up all organs of the body.

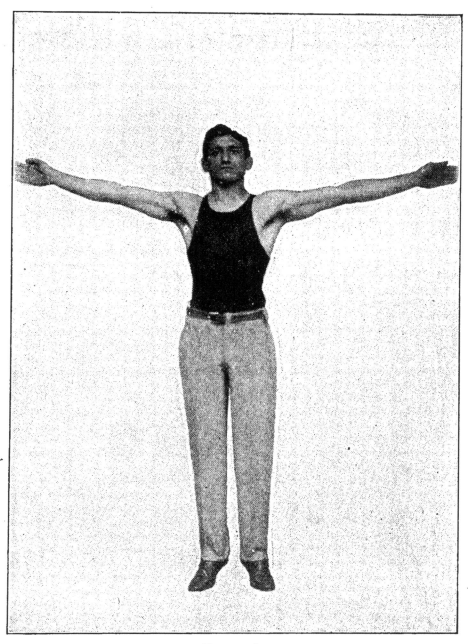

FIGURE 6.

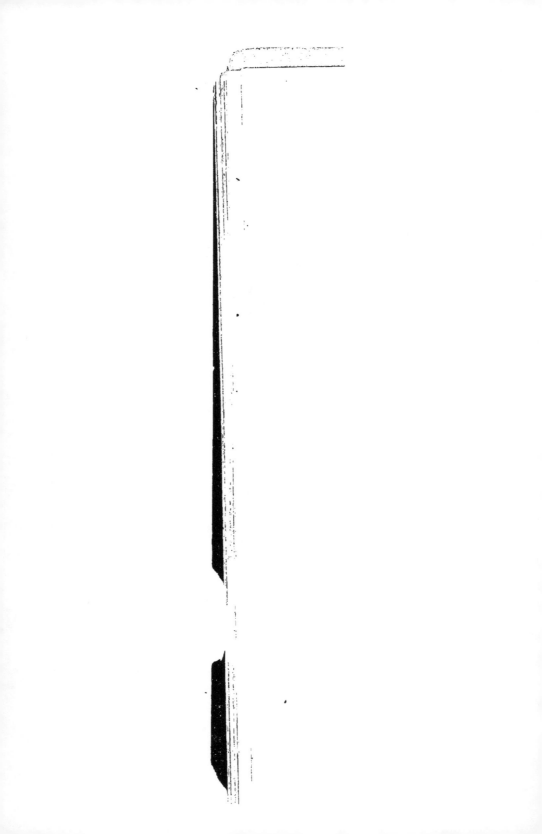

FOURTH EXERCISE.

The military commands used for the fourth exercise are:

1. Arm.

2. Exercise.

3. Shoulder.

4. Front.

5. Rear.

ARM.

1. Position as in Figure 1.

EXERCISE.

2. At the command *exercise,* raise the arms laterally, as in the first exercise.

SHOULDER.

3. Bend the arms so as to bring the hands above the shoulders and close to the neck.

Keep the upper arm horizontal.

The tips of the fingers should be placed lightly on the top of the shoulders.

See Fig. 8.

FRONT.

4. Keeping the arms at the same angle, force them to the front so that the elbows will be on a line with the chin, the hands being close to the side of the cheek.

The upper arm must be kept at the horizontal, as in the former movement.

See Fig. 9.

REAR.

5. Force the elbows to the rear as far as possible, the upper arm still retaining the horizontal.

See Fig. 10.

In this movement it will not be possible to get the arms very far to the rear, but the muscles will be strengthened by making the attempt, however unsuccessful.

Continue the exercise by alternating the front and rear movements, returning at the finish to the third position, and so back to attention.

Repeat the words *front* and *rear,* at the expiration of the movements, if commands are used.

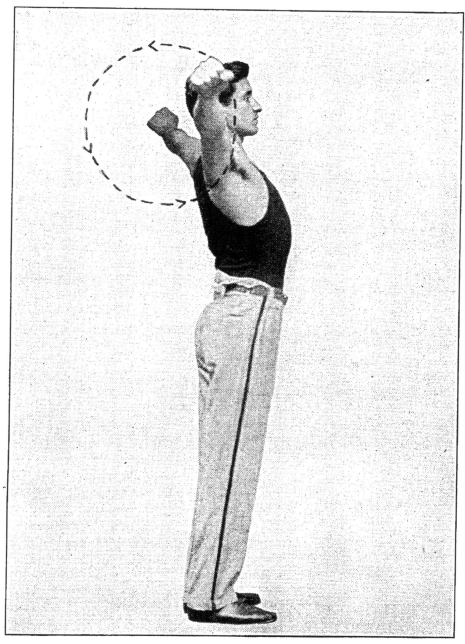

FIGURE 7.

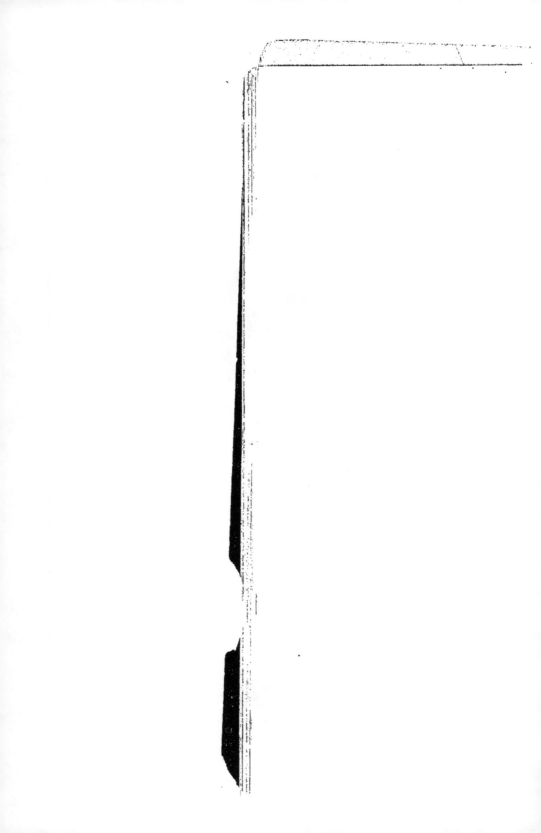

FIFTH EXERCISE.

The military commands used for the fifth exercise are:

1. Hand.

2. Exercise.

3. Close.

4. Open.

HAND.

1. Assume position as in Figure 1.

EXERCISE.

2. At the command *exercise,* raise the arms laterally, as in first exercise.

CLOSE.

3. Keeping the arms immovable, shut the hands with a quick, forcible movement, pressing the finger tips into the palm, the thumb being bent over the middle joint of the fingers.

Fig. 11 shows the correct angle of arms before closing the hands.

4. With arms in the same position, jerk open the
hand quickly, spreading the fingers and thumbs apart
as far as possible.

See Fig. 12.

Continue the exercise by rapidly opening and shut-
ting the hand.

Repeat the words *close, open,* if commands are used.

Between the movements there should be a slight
pause, but the movements themselves must be made
with the utmost rapidity.

Do not feel worried if you should become a little
sore after these exercises.

The best way to avoid stiffness of the muscles is to
commence quite moderately and finish with a sponge
bath, rubbing and kneading the muscles all over and
applying alcohol if needed.

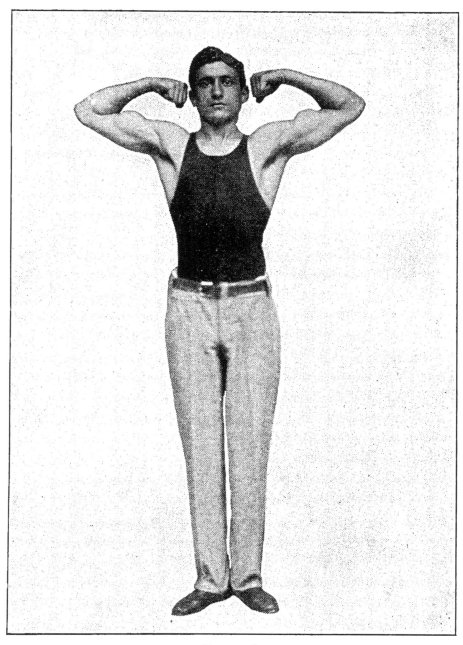

FIGURE 8.

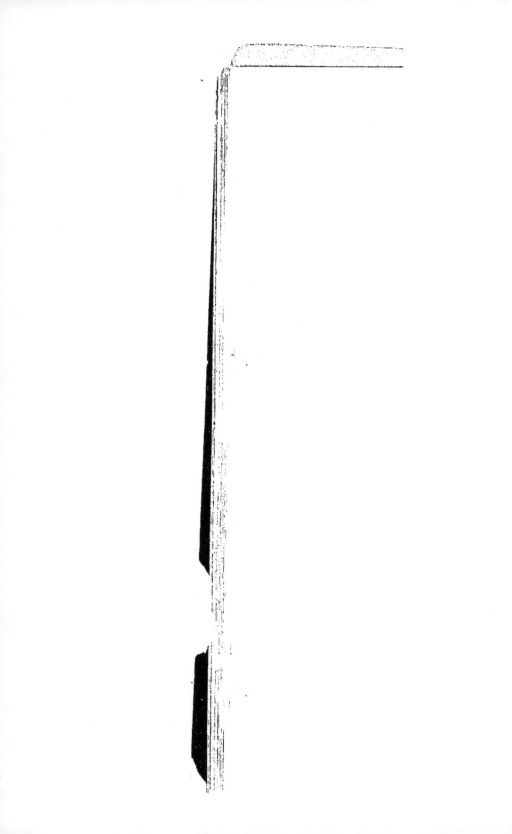

SIXTH EXERCISE.

The military commands used in the sixth exercise are:

1. Forearms vertical.
2. Raise.
3. Up.
4. Down.

FOREARMS VERTICAL.

1. Take position as in Figure 1.

RAISE.

2. At the command *raise,* bend the arms V-shape by elevating the forearms until nearly vertical.

Extend the fingers of each hand their full length and join them.

The palms of the hands should be turned toward each other.

Upper arm must only be inclined from the body sufficiently to permit forearm to be raised to the perpendicular.

The extended fingers and hand should be slightly inclined toward the side of the face.

See Fig. 13.

UP.

3. Thrust the hands forward with full force, extending the arms to their fullest length.

See Fig. 4.

DOWN.

4. Force the arms backward in an oblique direction and gradually allow them to fall by the sides.

See Fig. 1.

Continue the exercise by flexing the forearms and raising and lowering them as directed.

Repeat the words *raise, up, down,* if commands are used.

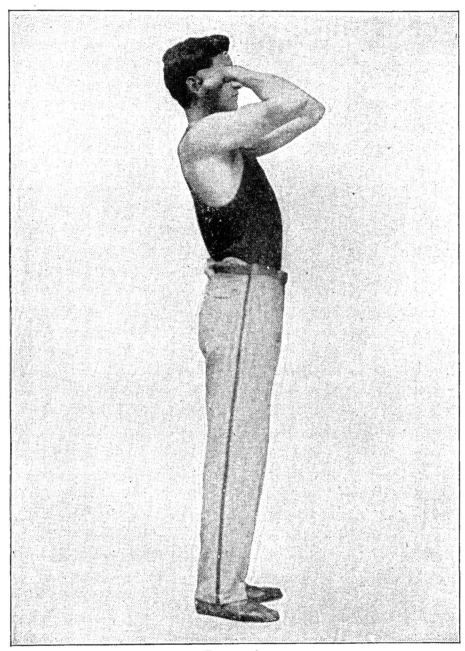

FIGURE 9.

SEVENTH EXERCISE.

The military commands used in the seventh exercise are:

1. Forearms horizontal.
2. Raise.
3. Front.
4. Rear.

FOREARMS HORIZONTAL.

1. Take position as in Figure 1.

RAISE.

2. At the command *raise,* elevate the forearms only so that they shall be at right angles to the body, the elbows being pressed backward only slightly, so as not to interfere with the horizontal line which must be retained by the forearms.

The hands may be kept either open or closed and extended in front, with backs down.

Avoid bringing the head forward in this exercise. The chest should be expanded to its fullest as the arms reach the limit of the backward motion. Remember in this movement that if a line be dropped perpendicularly in front of the body the chest should be the only point of contact.

See Fig. 14.

FRONT.

3. Thrust the arms forcibly to the front so that the whole arm shall be horizontal.

With the movement the hands should be turned with their backs uppermost.

The hands may be kept either open or closed, as may have been determined in the preceding movement.

The body should be swayed a little to the rear, keeping the feet firmly on the ground, the weight being transferred to the heel from the ball of the foot.

See Fig. 15.

REAR.

4. Bring the arms back quickly to the rear, forcing the elbows and shoulders backward as far as possible.

Keep the forearms at the horizontal.

Continue the exercise by alternating the rear and front movements, using full force with each change.

Repeat the words *front, rear,* if commands are used.

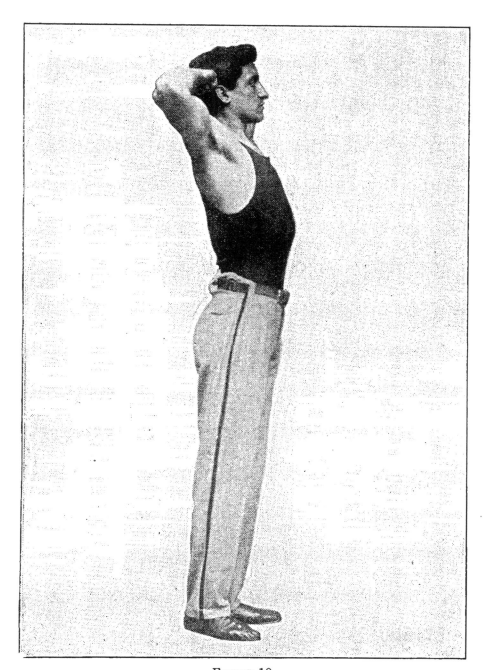

FIGURE 10.

EIGHTH EXERCISE.

The military commands used in the eighth exercise are:

1. Trunk.
2. Exercise.
3. Down.
4. Back.

TRUNK.

1. Take position as in Figure 1.

EXERCISE.

2. At the command *exercise,* raise the hands from the sides and place the palms on the hips.

Fingers to the front.

Thumbs to the rear.

Elbows pressed back.

See Fig. 16.

DOWN.

3. Bend the trunk forward at the hips.

Keep the head well up.

Shoulders pressed back.

Chest expanded and prominent.

Legs straight.

See Fig. 17.

BACK.

4. Raise the body upward and bend the trunk as · far to the rear as possible.

See Fig. 18.

In these movements do not hurry; exercise both movements (downward and backward) slowly, without bending the knees.

It is a good plan when first learning these movements to go through the exercises slowly until you can be sure of making each movement in a perfectly smooth and correct manner, when you can increase the speed.

To continue the exercise, repeat the words *down* and *back,* if commands are used, allowing plenty of time in each case.

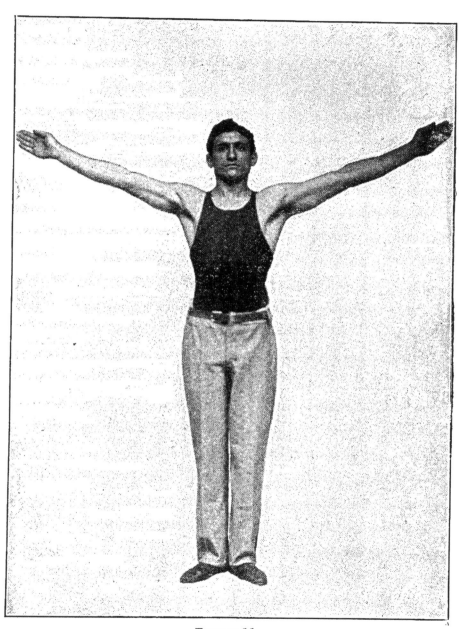

FIGURE 11.

NINTH EXERCISE.

The military commands used in the ninth exercise are:

1. Trunk.
2. Exercise.
3. Right.
4. Left.

TRUNK.

1. Take position as in Figure 1.

EXERCISE.

2. At the command *exercise,* bring the hands from the sides and place them on the hips, fingers to the front, thumbs to the rear, as in the eighth exercise.

RIGHT.

3. Bend the trunk to the right as far as possible.

Do not twist the body in making this movement. Face the front and let the trunk sway squarely to the side.

Both heels must be kept firmly fixed upon the ground, despite the tendency to raise one or other.

Keep the legs straight, and do not bend the knees even slightly.

LEFT.

4. Raise the body slowly and bend the trunk similarly to the left as far as possible.

Follow same directions as in former movement.

Execute both movements slowly.

To continue the exercise, repeat the words *right, left,* when commands are used.

See Fig. 19.

This exercise means a strain if long continued, and should be practiced carefully.

At its conclusion any slight feeling of strain should pass away quickly.

If it does not, then it is safe to suppose that you have gone beyond your strength, and the error should not be repeated.

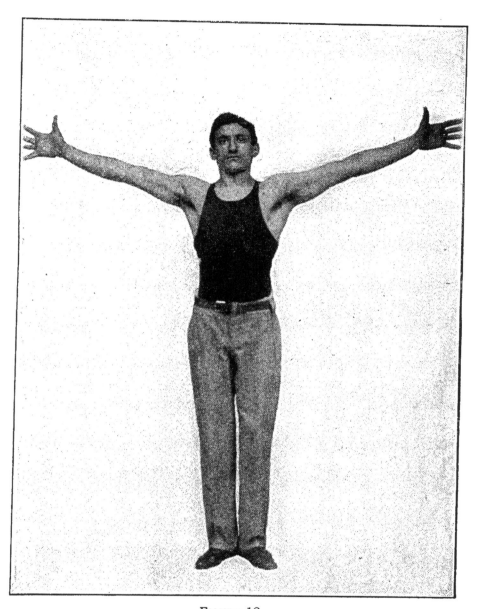

FIGURE 12.

TENTH EXERCISE.

The military commands used in the tenth exercise are:

1. Trunk.
2. Exercise.
3. Circle right (or left).

TRUNK.

1. Take position as in figure 1.

EXERCISE.

2. At the command *exercise,* raise the hands from the sides to the hips, fingers to the front, thumbs caught in the band of the trousers.

CIRCLE RIGHT.

1. Bend the trunk to the right, as in ninth exercise.

Circle toward the rear, so that body shall be in same position as in eighth exercise at the completion of the rearward movement.

See Fig. 20.

CIRCLE LEFT.

Continue circle to the left, so that body shall be in same position as in ninth exercise at the completion of the left movement.

Continue circle to the front, so that body shall be in same position as in eighth exercise at the end of the downward movement.

In other words, describe as large a circle as possible with the head and trunk without bending the knees or moving the feet.

To continue the exercise; repeat the word *circle,* with the completion of the movement, if commands are used.

Too much stress cannot be laid on the importance of concentrating the mind on each muscle affected by this exercise as it is being performed.

Your heart must be in your work.

Put your whole strength into each movement until the muscles ache, then pass on to the next exercise, but do not forget to relax the contraction at the end of the movement.

Until the muscles ache slightly they cannot develop to any great extent.

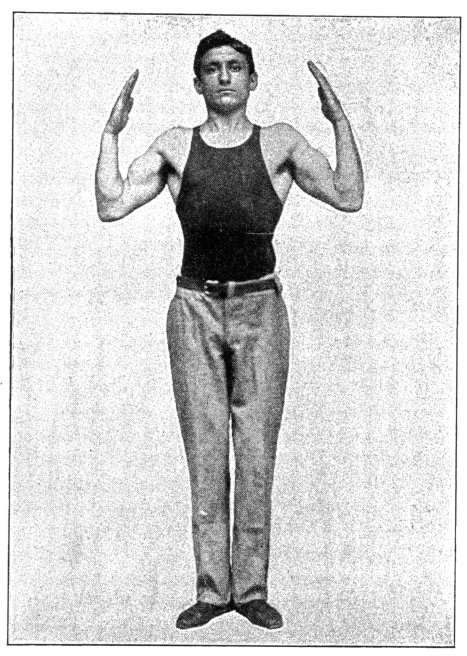

FIGURE 13.

ELEVENTH EXERCISE.

The military commands used in the eleventh exercise are:

1. Arms vertical.   Palms to the front.
2. Raise.
3. Down.
4. Up.

ARMS VERTICAL.

1. Take position as in Figure 1.

RAISE.

2. At the command *raise,* bring the arms upward from the sides until they are at full stretch directly above the head.

Do not at any time during the movement allow the arms to be bent.   They must be kept rigid and extended to their fullest length while accomplishing the sweep.

When the arms have been raised over the head the hands should be joined, with palms facing to the front, fingers pointed upward and thumbs locked, with right thumb in front.

Keep the shoulders pressed back.

See Fig. 21.

DOWN.

3. Bend the trunk forward at the hips and lower the arms so that the hands shall, if possible, touch the ground.

Keep the arms and knees straight.

See Fig. 22.

UP.

4. Straighten the body and swing the arms, extended to their full length, outward and upward to the vertical position.

Continue exercise by lowering and raising the hands, repeating the words *down, up,* at the end of each movement, if commands are used.

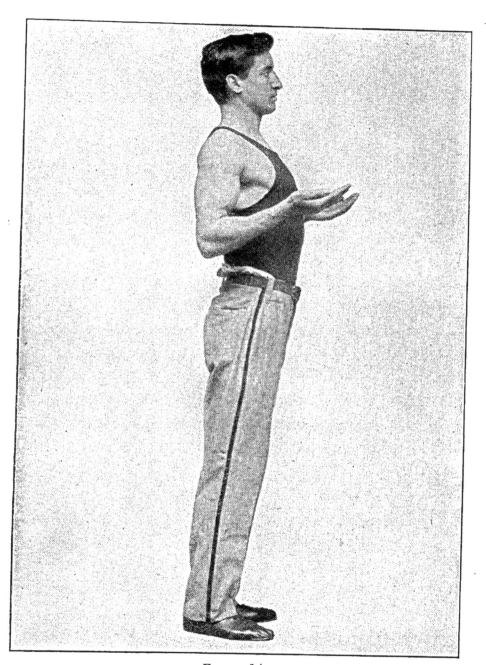

FIGURE 14.

TWELFTH EXERCISE.

The military commands used in the twelfth exercise are :

1. Arms forward. Palms down.
2. Raise.
3. Down.
4. Up.

ARMS FORWARD.

1. Take position as in Figure 1.

RAISE.

2. At the command *raise,* bring the arms from the sides upward to the front until they are horizontally extended to their full length and joined in front of the shoulders.

The palms must face downward.

Fingers extended and joined.

Thumbs under forefingers.

The arms should be raised not higher than, and in a line with, the shoulders.

See Fig. 23.

DOWN.

3. Bend the trunk forward at the hips as far as possible and with the movement swing the arms downward, backward and upward, so that at the end of the motion the hands are back of the shoulders and above them.

The hands need not be joined on being swung to the rear.

Keep the arms rigid.

Do not bend the knees.

The arms should be swung vertically, not horizontally, as in the second exercise.

See Fig. 24.

UP.

4. Straighten the body and swing the arms to the forward position.

Continue exercise by alternating the forward and backward movements.

Repeat the words *down, up,* if using commands.

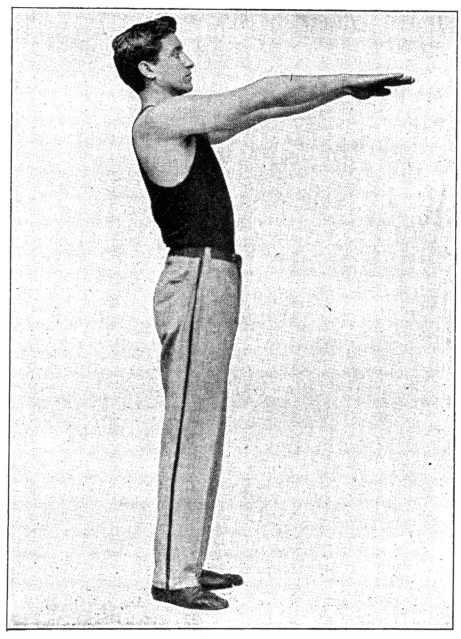

FIGURE 15.

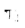

THIRTEENTH EXERCISE.

———

The military commands for the thirteenth exercise are:

1. Leg.
2. Exercise.
3. Half-bend.
4. Down.
5. Up.

LEG.

1. Take position as in Figure 1.

EXERCISE.

2. At the command *exercise,* raise the hands from the sides and place them on the hips, fingers to the front, thumbs to the rear, as in the eighth exercise.

HALF-BEND.

3. The thirteenth and fourteenth exercises are somewhat similar and the same commands—with one exception—are used in each. The word *half-bend* is

used as a preparatory to the ensuing movement, just as the word *full-bend* is used in the fourteenth exercise. No action accompanies the command, however; it is merely the signal to get ready for the movements that are to follow.

DOWN.

4. Lower the body by separating the knees and bending the legs as much as possible.

In this movement the heels must be kept firmly on the ground and must touch each other throughout the exercise.

Keep the back straight and the head erect.

See Fig. 25.

UP.

5. Raise the body by straightening the legs and closing the knees, resuming position as in eighth exercise.

Repeat several times without haste, using the words *down, up,* at the end of each movement for continuance of exercise, when commands are employed.

Observe carefully the instruction in this exercise and compare with the fourteenth.

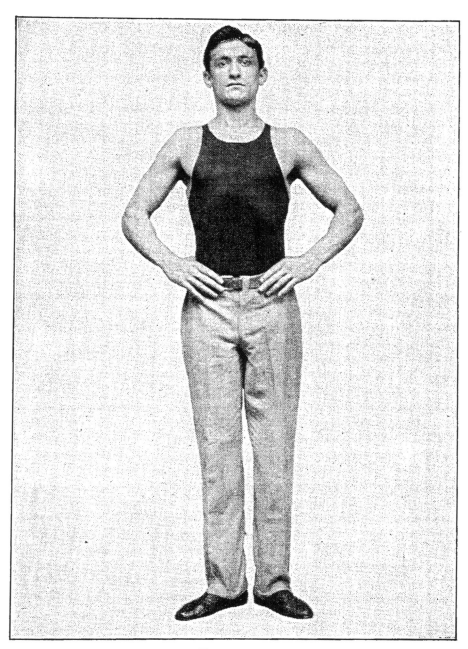

FIGURE 16.

FOURTEENTH EXERCISE.

The military commands used in the fourteenth exercise are:

1. Leg.
2. Exercise.
3. Full-bend.
4. Down.
5. Up.

LEG.

1. Take position as in Figure 1.

EXERCISE.

2. At the command *exercise,* raise the hands from the sides and place them on the hips, fingers to the front, thumbs to the rear, as in the eighth exercise.

FULL-BEND.

3. This military command is used to distinguish the fourteenth from the thirteenth exercise, as before explained. No action accompanies the word. It is a preparatory signal merely.

DOWN.

4. Lower the body to a sitting position by bending the legs and separating the knees, allowing the heels to be raised from the ground and the weight of the body to be thrown upon the balls of the feet.

Attention is directed to the important point of difference between this and the thirteenth exercise. In the preceding instance, the heels must be kept on the ground, while in this case the heels are raised, thus allowing the body to be bent much more than is possible in the thirteenth exercise.

Keep the back straight and vertical; the head and trunk should be erect.

See Fig. 26.

UP.

5. Raise the body by straightening the legs and bringing the knees together.

With the movement bring the heels again to the ground, transferring the weight of the body from the balls of the feet to the heels.

Repeat upward and downward movements slowly, using the words *down, up,* for continuance of exercise when commands are employed.

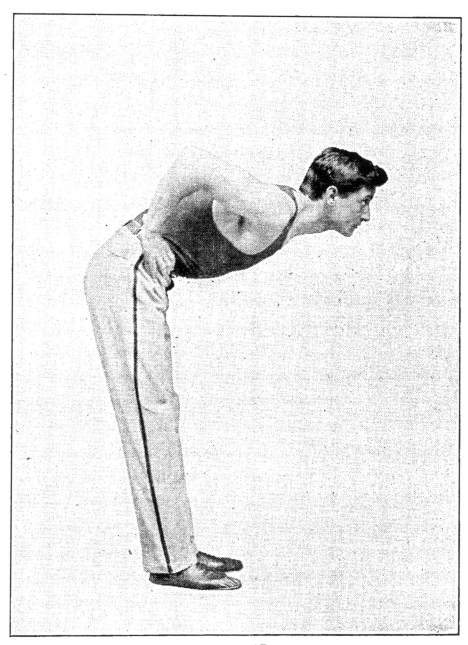

FIGURE 17.

FIFTEENTH EXERCISE.

———

· The military commands for the fifteenth exercise are:

1. Leg.
2. Exercise.
3. Left (or right).
4. Forward.
5. Rear, or Ground.

LEG.

1. Take position as in Figure 1.

EXERCISE.

2. At the command *exercise,* bring the hands from the sides and place them on the hips, fingers to the front, thumbs to the rear, as in the eighth exercise.

LEFT (OR RIGHT).

3. The words *left* or *right* are employed as preparatory signals to define the direction which the succeeding movements shall take.

No action accompanies the command.

FORWARD.

4. Supposing that it is decided to use the *left* movement: Raise the left foot from the ground and throw it slowly forward about fifteen inches.

Both legs must be kept straight.

Keep the toes turned outward.

The sole of the foot should be as nearly horizontal as possible, remembering not to bend the knee.

The body should be perfectly balanced on the right foot.

See Fig. 27.

REAR.

5. Bring the leg down and to the rear as far as possible, keeping the knees straight.

On the completion of the rearward swing the toe of the left foot should be on a line with the heel of the right foot, and the sole should be nearly horizontal.

Repeat forward and rearward movements slowly, using the words *forward, rear,* for the continuance of exercise when commands are employed.

The movement should be alternated with the right leg in action.

Fig. 28 shows the rearward action of the right leg.

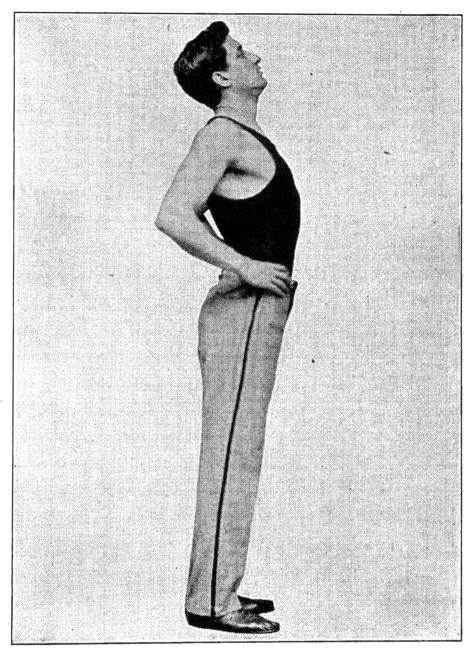

FIGURE 18.

GROUND.

When the balancing on one foot can be accomplished successfully, follow the command *forward* with the command *ground*.

Throw the entire weight of the body forward by rising on the ball of the right foot.

Advance and place the left foot firmly on the ground.

The left heel should be thirty inches from the right foot.

Advance the right leg quickly to the *forward* position.

Return to original position and repeat.

When using commands the word *ground* should be employed when the right and left legs are in the position of *forward*.

Thus: *Left forward, ground, right forward, ground, right rear, ground, left rear, ground,* and then continue *left forward, ground, etc.*

This is an excellent exercise for the development of the lower limbs, and any one who regularly includes this movement among the other exercises will surely strengthen and beautify this part of the muscular system. Walking will also strengthen the legs; indeed, walking is perhaps the best of all exercises that could be prescribed.

No other has its all-round merits or is quite its equal in value; but notwithstanding its great value it is not sufficient if all the attainable strength and symmetry of the limbs is desired.

The setting-up exercises must be added to it.

It must be remembered, however, by those who wish to possess strong legs, that the lower limbs can be developed much more speedily if the upper part of the body is not neglected.

It would be unwise to select this fifteenth exercise and say: "I will practice this only." Do not, forget the necessity for strong lungs in the desire for strong legs. They go together. Make no selections, but practice all the exercises.

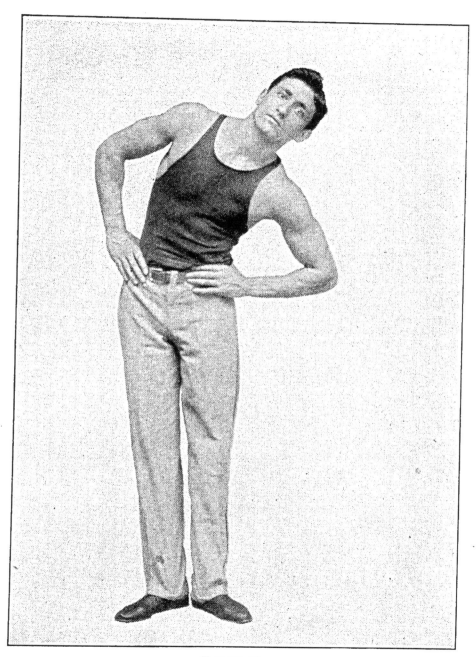

FIGURE 19.

SIXTEENTH EXERCISE.

The military commands used in the sixteenth ex-
cise are:

1. Leg.

2. Exercise.

3. Up.

4. Up.

LEG.

1. Take position as in Figure 1.

EXERCISE.

2. At the command *exercise,* bring the hands from
the sides to the hips, fingers to the front, thumbs to
the rear, as in eighth exercise.

UP.

3. Raise the left leg to the front, bending and elevating the knee as much as possible, and keeping the leg

from the knee to the instep vertical, with the toes depressed.

Keep the body straight.

UP.

4. Replace the left foot and raise the right leg as prescribed for the left.

See Fig. 29.

Execute these movements slowly at first, then gradually increase to the cadence of double time.

Alternate the movements of right and left foot.

When commands are used, repeat the word *up* when the right and left legs are alternately in position.

Continue this exercise until the muscles of the legs are thoroughly tired. If the resistance is too strong there is danger of becoming "muscle-bound"—an inflexible condition of the msucles which incapacitates them for any quick or graceful movements.

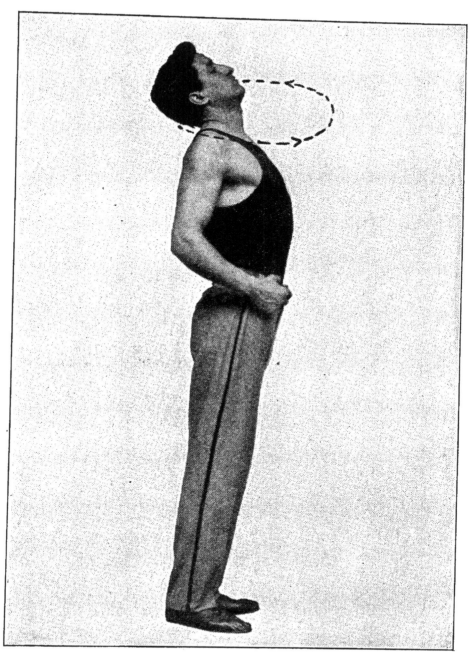

FIGURE 20.

SEVENTEENTH EXERCISE.

———

The military commands used in the seventeenth exercise—the last of the setting-up exercises—are:

1. Foot.
2. Exercise.
3. Up.
4. Down.

FOOT.

1. Take position as in Figure 1.

EXERCISE.

2. At the command *exercise*, bring the hands from the sides to the hips, fingers to the front, thumbs to the rear, as in the eighth exercise.

UP.

3. Raise the body upon the toes.

Do not bend the knees.

Keep the heels together.

See Fig. 30.

DOWN.

4. Lower the body slowly till the heels touch the ground.

Alternate the upward and downward movements slowly several times.

If using commands repeat the words *up, down,* to indicate that the exercise is to be continued.

It is sometimes the rule in the military school to omit the commands when the exercises are well understood. The instructor simply gives the commands as prescribed, then adds: *Continue the exercise,* wherefore the motions to be repeated are continuously exercised until the command *halt.*

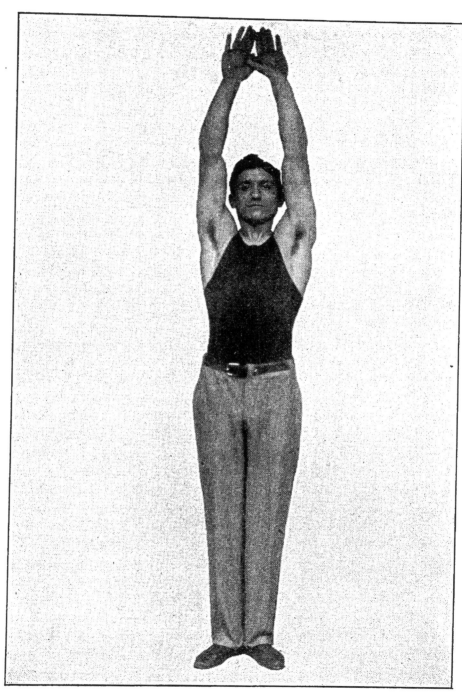

FIGURE 21.

GENERAL HINTS.

It is to be presumed that all who practice these set_ting-up exercises are in quest not only of strong muscles, but of a sound, healthy body. But something beyond physical culture is necessary for this.

Life is nothing more than a constant process of building up and breaking down of body tissues, so that a man is weak or strong, sickly or healthy, according as there is more of the breaking-down process going on, or more of the building-up. To be strong and healthy he must be doing more building up, and nothing is so essential to this object as good food and good digestion.

A good digestion means good teeth for the mastication of food, a good heart, blood vessels and blood, so as to give proper saliva, gastric juice, intestinal juice, and a healthy liver, and a good nervous system, so as to properly regulate the process of digestion.

Good teeth are absolutely essential. They should always be kept clean. Brush them daily. Rinse the mouth frequently. Consult a dentist at regular periods to guard against defective teeth.

Never bolt your food, but always chew it carefully. Take time to eat your meals. The more time that is spent in chewing, the less is required for digestion. Never eat when tired. Never eat immediately before active work.

Do not smoke, for it depresses the heart.

Do not drink, because it at first excites the heart and strains the blood vessels and afterward produces just the opposite effect, both of which interfere with digestion in healthy persons.

Do not eat while laboring under excitement of any kind, whether it be of joy, sorrow or anger, for all alike affect the heart so as to retard or prevent digestion.

Keep the bowels open, for if this is not done a part of the contents of the bowels is absorbed into the blood and acts as a poison upon the brain and whole nervous system, and thus deranges digestion.

Eat little or nothing if not hungry.

Never overfeed; it is harmful.

Eat your meat either roasted or broiled in an oven or pot.

Recollect that all that interferes with digestion,

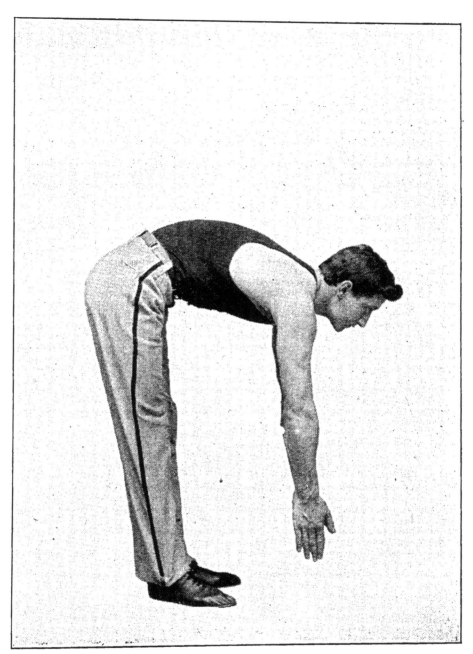

FIGURE 22.

eventually causes impoverished blood, and this leads to starvation of the digestive organs, poor digestion and inevitable loss of strength, sickness and death.

Water is one of the chief ingredients of food. The body could not thrive without it, and is necessarily not at its best when too little is taken.

Men who have made experiments in fasting find that they have been able to keep their fast from ten days to two weeks longer when they drink plenty of water.

Besides this, water is a great aid to digestion because it stimulates the flow of the gastric juice and puts some parts of the stomach contents into solution so that they are better prepared for the absorptive process of digestion.

Water flushes the kidneys and thus helps wonderfully in the excretion of those poisonous substances formed by the breaking-down process of the body.

It is an excellent thing, therefore, to drink water before, during, and after meals.

A goblet of water, taken before breakfast, does several things: It passes through the stomach into the small intestines in a continuous and uninterrupted flow. It partly distends the stomach. It thins and washes out into the gut most of the mucus. It wakes up, so to speak, the whole alimentary tract, and gives it a morning's exercise and washing.

The beneficial effects of a drink of water before breakfast may account for the desire 'for water at this time of the day, particularly on rising. How often we find that when we are very hungry we want a drink before beginning to eat.

Moderately cold water taken into the stomach chills locally; it stimulates to contraction and produces a re-action. A warm, healthy glow succeeds the contrac-tion due to the cold. The clean member is in excellent condition to receive food, which now comes in direct contact with the bare gastric wall. A copious flow of digestive juice is the result, and the food, not being covered with mucus, digestion is easy and rapid, for it takes place under the most favorable conditions and in a minimum time.

Most of the repair of the body takes place during sleep, that is, wear and tear is made good and a new supply of force is accumulated for expenditure during the next waking period. Hence sleep is very neces-sary to good health and strength.

It is just as important to sleep well as to eat well. Loss of sleep is as wearing as loss of food. Expe-rience has taught that one-third of adult life should

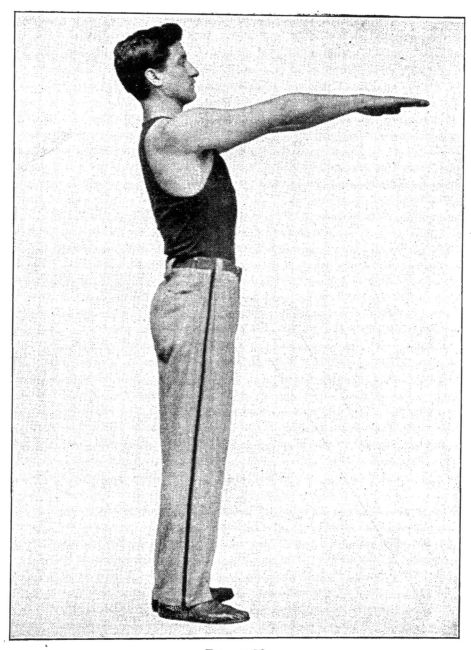

FIGURE 23.

be spent in sleep—in other words, eight hours out of every twenty-four.

It is better for the health to retire at 9 p. m. than at 11, and the following is the reason, and it is a good one:

The "early-to-bed-and-early-to-rise" man gets just as many extra hours of sunlight as the number of hours he goes to bed before the accustomed time. It is plain, therefore, that with the increased benefit of longer sunshine, he should have better health than when retiring late at night.

But it is also the refreshing spirit that is infused by early rising and the observing of quiet nature that is beneficial, influencing the behavior during the balance of the day.

A volume may be written to point out the many ways in which early rising does good, but these few examples must suffice, while the reader is advised to try it and think out the remaining benefits for himself. He will find new ones almost daily.

A man may feel stronger after taking a drink of spirits, but it is only artificial strength; when the effect passes away it leaves him in a weaker state. Whisky cures many ailments, but kills the patient. "He that is deceived is not wise."

The best treatment for biliousness is plenty of hard work to the point of free perspiration. This is particularly true if the work is done in the fresh, open air.

The would-be athlete should adopt at the beginning of his work a well-regulated and scientific system.

The following programme will be found especially useful:

1. Breakfast at 7 a. m., dinner at 12 m., supper at 6 p. m.

2. Chew food well—the stomach has no teeth.

3. Eat nothing between meals.

4. Never drink intoxicants.

5. Do not use tobacco in any form.

6. Live in open air as much as possible, at least three hours daily.

7. Always breathe through the nose and breathe deeply.

8. Keep neck, legs and arms well covered.

9. Exercise regularly every day.

10. Run on toes one-half mile daily.

11. Do not take too violent exercise.

12. Do not wear tight belts or coats fitting tightly over chest.

Every man should have this programme pasted up

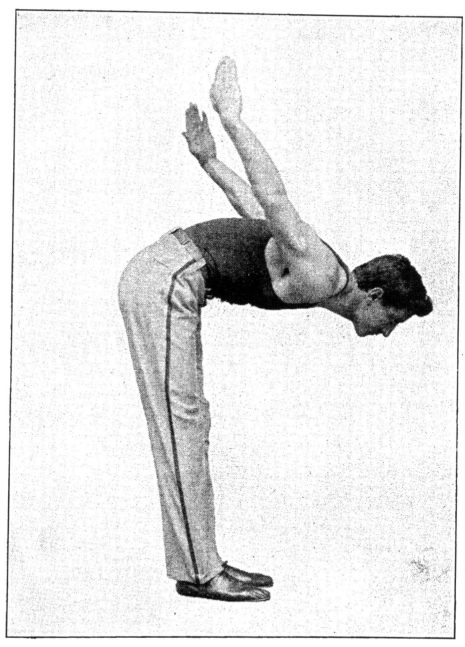

FIGURE 24.

in his room and follow it out religiously if he wants to train himself thoroughly.

Learn to do these things well and you will be on the high road to successful physical development.

THE HORIZONTAL BAR.

Many who practice the setting-up exercises may desire some more strenuous form of physical culture, and a word on the subject of gymnastics may be useful.

Perhaps of all gymnastic apparatus, the horizontal bar is the simplest. Any one with ingenuity can rig up one for himself and immediately have at his disposal one of the most important appurtenances of a well-equipped gymnasium.

No part of the body goes without exercise while the gymnast uses the bar. The muscles of the legs, arms, wrists, hands, chest, back and abdomen, alike receive the greatest possible benefit.

To HANG ON THE BAR BY THE HANDS.—Place the bar so that when standing flat on the feet, and stretching the arms well above the head, it shall be about six inches above the tips of the fingers; then jump up, and by passing the hands over it toward the back, lay hold of it and grasp it firmly, letting the thumbs be on the same side as the fingers, and the knuckles as far upward as possible, grasping it firmly, without any fear of not being able to retain your hold very long, as that is sure to come by practice.

Therefore, at first suspend yourself as long as convenient without tiring yourself, yet after a time you should so hang as long as possible; and by the continual practice of this, the most simple of all exer-- cises, the strength of the arms and hands is greatly developed.

Though not fatiguing at first, it becomes much more so the longer the body is suspended, and it is stated that a soldier once held himself by the hands for forty-two minutes, while many others have been known to thus suspend themselves for thirty-five minutes.

TO HANG BY THE HANDS.—Stand under the bar with the face toward its length, and in jumping up to grasp it place one hand on either side of it, and proceed as stated in the last exercise.

Jump up as in the first exercise, but grasp the bar with the arms crossed about halfway between the elbows and the wrists, and letting the face come between the arms so as to look between them, at the same time keeping the body perfectly straight by not allowing it to turn either to the right or to the left, according to whichever arm is underneath.

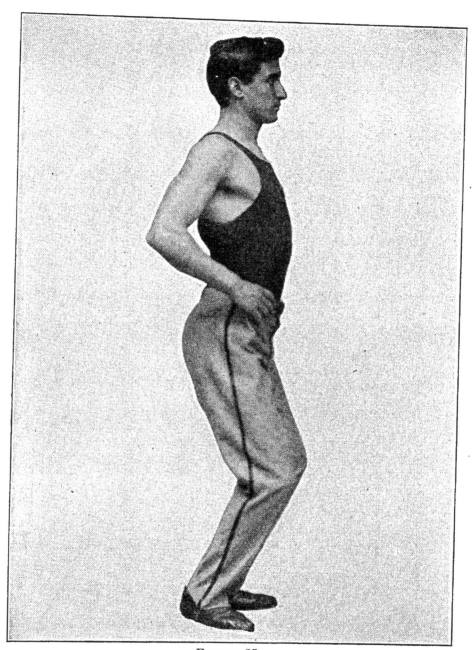

FIGURE 25.

BREASTING THE BAR.—This exercise is nothing more than the pulling up of the body as high as the arms will allow.

It is done by hanging on the bars by the hands and gradually raising the body, by bending the arms at the elbows, until the breast is as high as the bar, then steadily lowering yourself again.

It should be repeated at least three times, and if not able to succeed in doing it the first time of trying do not despair, for on the being able to effect this exercise likewise depends the being able to accomplish many other; besides which, it tends greatly to strengthen the muscles of the arms and wrist.

TO TOUCH THE BAR WITH THE FEET.—Hang on the bar as before described, and, with a gradual motion, bring the legs up toward it; bend the knees, and pass them between the arms under the bar together with the toes, which must be pressed against it.

A slight swing might be used at first, if not able to bring up the legs without; but it is improper to do so, as, in all exercises where the legs are to be brought up, it ought to be done entirely through the muscular force of the arms.

TO HANG BY THE TOES.—Proceed as in the last, and, instead of placing the feet under the bar, hitch them over it, keeping the toes pointed toward the ground as much as possible.

Let go your hands, and gradually allow your body to hang straight down by alternately catching hold of your clothes until you are more expert, which you will be after trying it a few times.

But the most difficult part of this exercise is to be able to replace your hands on the bars.

To do so, pull yourself up by catching hold of your clothes, using your hands alternately in so doing; but if not able to, and the distance be not too great, un-hitch the toes and drop to the ground on the hands, letting the feet come down lightly.

THE PANCAKE.—Place the bar about two feet above the head of the gymnast when standing on the ground, and proceed as described in the last, and when the body has been swung nearly as high as the bar, let go your hands (the farther the gymnast springs from it the greater the effect), and after bringing them smartly together, renew your hold of the bar and continue to swing each time the exercise is to be repeated, which should be at least three times before allowing the feet to touch the ground.

It is a difficult exercise to beginners, but very soon mastered.

It must be borne in mind that on letting go the bar the gymnast must not do so as if he were trying to carry himself back from it as far as possible, but a

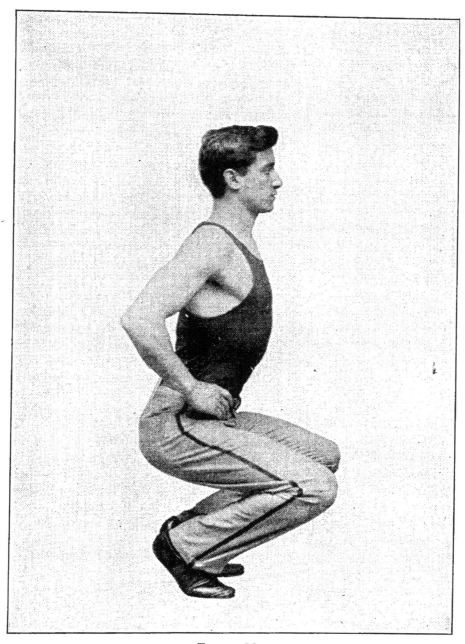

FIGURE 26.

slight forward spring must be given to enable him (if possible) to bring his hands together close to, if not just above, the bar.

THE PLYMOUTH.—Bring the legs through, and in carrying them over the bar let them be a little bent, then, bending the body well back, and turning the head back as far as possible, *i.e.,* the face toward the ground, and the farther you look along the ground the better, whereby the body is the better kept in 'that position, and which enables the exercise to be more easily done; raise the body up by the aid of your arms; then, when the bar is a little over the seat, by bending the legs more over it, which act as a sort of leverage to the body, you will be enabled to bring it over and assume a sitting posture.

But your own judgment must be used as to the best time to do so, for, when the bar touches the center of the back, the arms must do the remainder of the work, but do not pull yourself too far over the bar, otherwise, in assuming the sitting posture, a beginner is very likely to fall forward, which would not be very pleasant for his arms; but should a mishap occur, it will be well for him to give a slight spring forward and alight on the ground in front of the bar.

THE HINDOO PUNISHMENT, OR MUSCLE GRIND.—Sit on the bar and sink down, but letting the arms slip, one at a time first backward over the bar, when the hands can either be clasped across the chest, or grasp

a belt, which may be worn round the waist, if pre-
ferred; then, moving the legs and body to and fro
with a stronger impetus with the legs, carry the body
round the bar, which motion must be repeated, on the
body falling over, every time the gymnast wishes to go
round.

This should not be more than three times at first,
owing to the friction and rubbing which the arms will
get until 'more used to it, and until such is the case
they will be very red and tender after each practice—
so much so, that the gymnast will not like to repeat it
for a day or two; but that must not be noticed too
much, as the oftener the muscles are thus exercised
the less will be the notice taken of the results in future.

This exercise is reversed by carrying the legs and
body up in front instead, thereby revolving round the
other way, but the arms remain the same; and, in this,
as in many other exercises before mentioned, the legs
must be made good use of.

The gymnast, when perfect in either way, but generally the first, would do well to try how many times
he can go round, or at least from twelve to twenty
times.

THE USE OF FLYING RINGS.

The advantage which the flying rings have over the
bar is that, from their being suspended from the ceil-
ing, they can be used almost everywhere, even in a

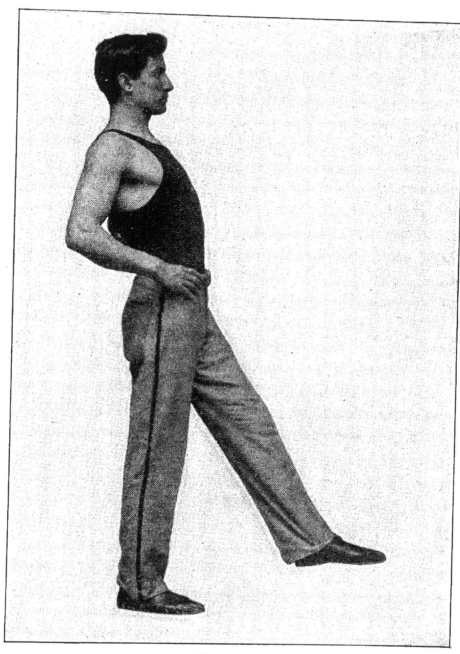

FIGURE 27.

passage about three feet wide, room to swing to and fro being the chief requisite.

There is scarcely a part of the body, from the hands to the feet, that is not brought into use by practicing upon the rings, and the effects of being carried backward and forward in the swing being so well known to every one, what must therefore be the additional benefits to be derived from suspending the body by the hands while being thus swayed to and fro.

Though the exercises are not so various upon the rings as upon the bar, still gymnasts will be generally found practicing upon them oftener.

The gymnast should start this exercise with simple arm movement, such as taking hold of the rings with his hands and gradually drawing himself up to his chin, and then letting himself down to arm's length.

This should be done slowly and repeatedly, from six to eight times in succession. In the course of several weeks he will find that he can do it twenty times with the same ease that he did his six or eight turns when he first began.

This exercise brings into play, particularly, the muscles of the arms.

If this work is completely mastered I would advise what commonly goes by the name of "breast up." There are two ways of accomplishing this trick. One is with the single grip and the other is with the double grip.   There is all the difference in the world between the single and double grip.

The single grip is by far the most difficult of the two, and I advise particularly against its use.   With the double grip it is altogether different.   You place your hands on the rings and allow them to rest almost halfway across the wrists.   You will find that in the course of time you will be able to do it with very little exertion.

To make this trick plainer I will add a few words: You must place, as I have already described, your hands above the rings, and then draw yourself up so as to have the hands even with the shoulders, which is not very easy; then you turn the rings out, in order to allow your shoulders to come between the ropes. Now draw the rings toward you, press until you get up at arm's length, and the trick is done.

When the trick is done with the single grip a great deal of weight must be supported by the fingers alone. When it is done with the double grip the whole hand and also the wrist are used, and thus the labor is divided.

This trick should be thoroughly studied and mastered, and when that is done the beginner will be amply rewarded.   He will have far less trouble and exercise less strength in doing the more difficult tricks, such as the forward horizontal, back horizontal, hand balance, stationary and swinging; the half-arm balance, back

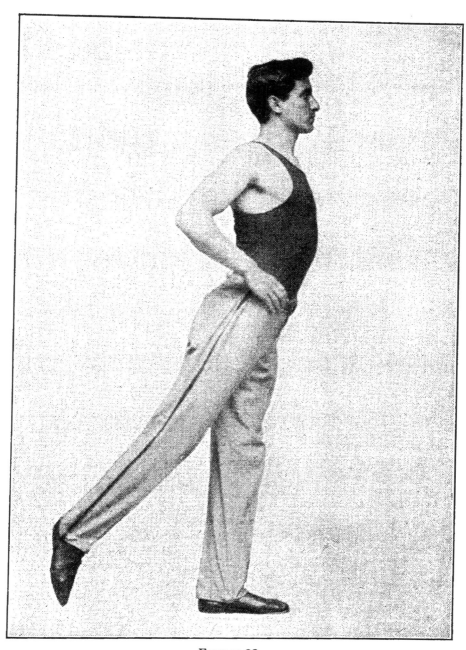

FIGURE 28.

snap, stationary and swing and double disjoint, slow revolve and many others too numerous to mention.

I consider it best to use the double grip in studying the rings, as I find that it enables the performer not only to do all these tricks better, but also with much more ease and grace.

One thing a beginner should never lose sight of. He should be careful to finish his tricks as well and neatly as possible, so as to make them graceful and appear easy to the spectator.

He must be precise in every movement, not a second too long nor too short. He should start in and leave off at the precise moment.

To beginners I would say do all your tricks with style and finish, for however simple a trick may be, if it is perfectly done it will be a pleasure to the beholder. But, on the contrary, if the most difficult trick is not well done it is a failure, and would better not have been attempted.

A beginner will find that the rings are about as hard as any apparatus in the gymnasium.

But no gymnasium work is easy, and perseverance is the key of success. If the first effort is a failure the fifth or sixth may not be. My advice is to work persistently and never lose heart.

I have already described the process of training for the rings, and now I will tell how some of the tricks are performed.

The back horizontal is one of the prettiest that I know of. In this trick the performer takes hold of the rings, and throws his legs into the air until he is in the position of a man standing on his hands. Slowly the body is lowered until it is held out straight with the face downward and the arms extended downward.

The front horizontal is much more difficult to most performers, but with me it is easier. The beginner should start by hanging at arm's length. Then he should throw the head well back and draw his legs and body up until a horizontal is reached. This should be done at first with a forward snap.

The swinging back snap is simply a breast-up done backward and with a throw. The performer rests on his palms at arm's length. This trick does not require so much strength as knack. It is not hard to learn and needs confidence. The beginner should do it first without a swing.

The swinging hand balance requires first breast-up. When you are up at the forward end of the rings throw your feet up and strike a balance with your legs over your head.

The learner should first balance on his hands on the floor with his feet against the wall. Gradually he should draw away from the support in order to gain independence.

On the rings it should be learned without the swing.

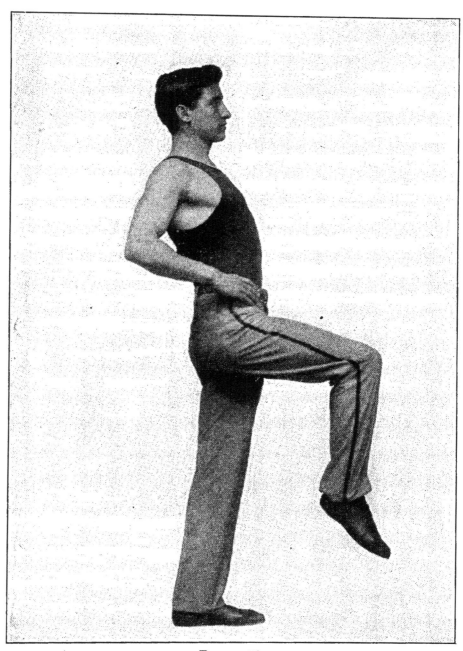

FIGURE 29.

When this is mastered a short swing should be tried. Gradually increase the swing until in the air and in motion the performer is perfectly at home. This trick requires nerve, confidence and knack.

The half-arm balance consists of resting the weight of the body on the forearm, which is passed through the rings below the elbow, throwing the feet up and stopping at a balance. This trick requires little prae-tice, and always attracts attention. But unless the rings are held in one place the arms are likely to be hurt.

In making the slow revolve the performer should first do the breast-up, keeping the arms at full length. Gradually he should lower the body to the forward horizontal position, and then complete the revolution until the original position is reached.

A SPECIMEN TRAINING TABLE.

The training table is a very old institution. In olden times the gladiators were kept on a strict diet for weeks before their contests.

Even stricter were the regulations imposed upon the athletes of the English universities within the last century, but to-day, while the training table is looked upon as absolutely necessary for the development of the athlete, its regulations are more lenient and alto-gether better, since scientists have done much to prove

the high value of certain foods which were heretofore
looked upon as injurious.

All the athletic teams in our great universities have
their special training tables.   The members of the
teams are allowed to eat nowhere else, for here their
diet is regulated by their trainers, and each man is
therefore allowed to eat only those things most beneficial in developing him physically.

A special corps of cooks is employed to prepare the
food and a special diet table is prescribed by the head
trainer.

Some trainers go so far as to claim that one-half
the success of a 'team depends upon the training table.
The following may be taken as a fair training table
for amateur athletes:

MONDAY.

Breakfast.—Oatmeal, codfish cakes, milk, bread
butter.

Dinner.—Beefsteak, potatoes, green corn, bread and
butter, rice pudding, fruits in season.

Supper.—Cold meat, milk, bread and butter, prunes.

TUESDAY.

Breakfast.—Pettijohn, lamb chops, milk, wheat
cakes, bread and butter.

Dinner.—Roast beef, potatoes, macaroni, peas,
bread and butter, bread pudding, fruits in season.

Supper.—Cold roast beef, crackers and cheese, milk,
bread and butter.

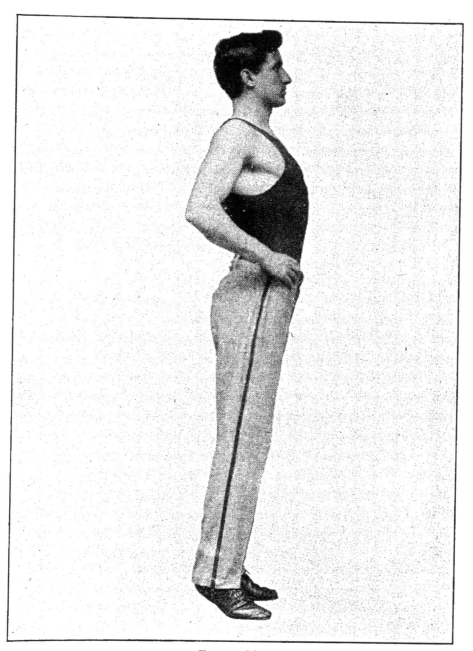

FIGURE 30.

WEDNESDAY.

Breakfast.—Oatmeal, corn bread and butter, poached eggs, milk.

Dinner.—Roast mutton, potatoes, tomatoes, bread and butter, tapioca pudding, fruits in season.

Supper.—Cold mutton, buttered toast, prunes, cocoa.

THURSDAY.

Breakfast.—Shredded wheat, calf's liver, creamed potatoes, brown bread, milk.

Dinner.—Beefsteak, mashed potatoes, beets, peas, bread and butter, Indian pudding, fruits in season.

Supper.—Oyster stew, crackers, bread and butter.

FRIDAY.

Breakfast.—Oatmeal, codfish cakes, milk, bread and butter.

Dinner.—Steak halibut, mashed potatoes, peas, tomatoes, bread and butter, cup custard.

Supper.—Corn fritters, potato cakes, bread and butter, prunes, cocoa.

SATURDAY.

Breakfast.—Oatmeal, scrambled eggs, milk, bread and butter.

Dinner.—Beefstew, potatoes, green corn, bread and butter, cottage pudding.

Supper.—Baked beans, bread and butter, weak tea, prunes.

SUNDAY.

Breakfast.—Oatmeal, rolls, boiled eggs, wheat cakes, cup of coffee.

Dinner.—Rib roast, mashed potatoes, peas, tomatoes, green corn, bread and butter, ice cream, fruits in season.

Supper.—Cold tongue, hashed brown potatoes, weak tea, crackers, bread and butter, jelly or jam.

In making out this diet table I have avoided the general use of coffee and tea and recommend their very infrequent use simply to lend variety to the diet.

THE END.

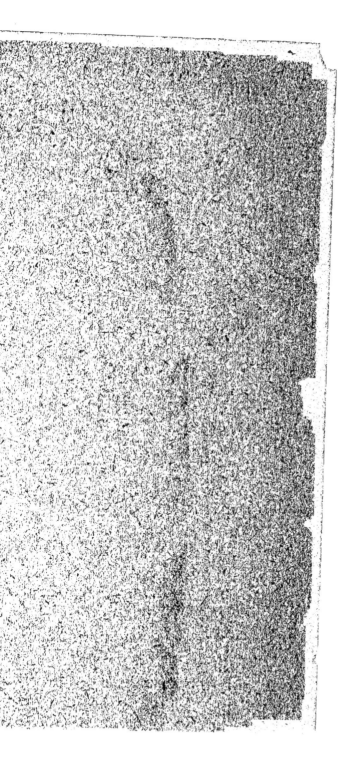

Diamond Hand-Book Series

A monthly publication devoted to good literature. By subscription, $1 75 per year (postpaid). Aug., 1902. Street & Smith, 238 William St., N. Y.

NO. 11

Information
FOR
Everybody

OUR new series of **Diamond Hand Books** cannot be equaled. All the books contained in this line have been written by authors who have given the subjects long and careful study. The following is a list of those which have been published, more will follow:

1—Sheldon's Letter Writer. L. W. SHELDON.

2—Guide to Love, Courtship and Marriage. } GRACE SHIRLEY.

3—Women's Secrets or How to be Beautiful. } GRACE SHIRLEY.

4—Sheldon's Guide to Etiquette. L. W. SHELDON.

5—Physical Health Culture. PROF. FOURMEN.

6—Frank Merriwell's Book of Athletic Development. } BURT L. STANDISH.

7—National Dream Book. MME. CLAIRE ROUGEMONT.

8—Zingara Fortune Teller. BY A GIPSY QUEEN.

For sale at all newsdealers.
If ordered by mail 4 cents must be added for postage.

STREET & SMITH, *Publishers*
NEW YORK.